DISCLAIMER

The nutritional recommendations and recipes in this book are meant solely for informative reasons. They are not meant to replace the counsel, diagnosis, or care of a qualified medical expert. If you have any doubts about a medical condition or dietary requirements, you should always see your physician or another trained healthcare expert.

All reasonable efforts have been taken by the author and publisher to ensure that the information contained in this book is correct as of the date of publication. Recommendations may alter, though, as medical knowledge is always changing. When using any of the recipes or instructions found here, the user assumes all liability and assumes no risk, whether personal or otherwise. People who have certain dietary requirements or medical issues should speak with a healthcare provider for personalized guidance. The given recipes are only ideas; you may need to adjust them to suit your own nutritional needs, tastes, and tolerances.

When you use this book, you agree to release the publisher, the author, and their representatives from any liability for any claims, damages, liabilities, costs, or expenditures resulting from your use of the book.

TABLE OF CONTENTS

ABOUT THE BOOK

The Chronic Fatigue Syndrome Diet Cookbook is an invaluable tool for anyone attempting to navigate the intricacies of managing Chronic Fatigue Syndrome (CFS) with food. Understanding the critical role diet plays in reducing symptoms and improving general health, the cookbook covers the unique dietary requirements and difficulties that individuals with CFS encounter.

Its importance stems primarily from the thorough understanding it offers of CFS itself, including its symptoms, diagnosis, and how diet directly influences these aspects.

The cookbook also empowers readers to make informed dietary choices that can positively affect their daily lives by describing the impact of nutrition on CFS symptoms and emphasizing the need for balanced meals that are specifically designed to manage CFS symptoms. It also provides useful insights into essential nutrients and foods to include or avoid.

In addition, the cookbook provides helpful advice on how to plan and prepare meals so that people can simply incorporate these dietary guidelines into their daily routines. Each section of the cookbook, which includes everything from time-saving meal preparation tips to healthy cooking techniques that preserve essential nutrients, is made to make it easier for people to maintain a nutritious diet even with the difficulties that come with CFS.

The cookbook's main attraction is its abundance of recipes, which are carefully designed to accommodate a range of lifestyles and dietary constraints. Whether you're making hearty dinners, satisfying lunches, nourishing breakfasts, or healthy snacks and desserts, every recipe focuses on taste and nutrition. What's more, special considerations like handling dietary restrictions and modifying recipes for weight control are included, further highlighting the cookbook's practicality and inclusivity.

Answering frequently asked questions and addressing common issues, the cookbook offers insightful guidance on managing food sensitivities and allergies so that readers can confidently make dietary choices that support their health goals. It also offers invaluable advice on navigating fatigue-related challenges in cooking, maintaining balance during flare-ups, and providing useful tips for grocery shopping and meal preparation on low-energy days.

The cookbook also empowers people to maintain their dietary needs while having a fulfilling social life. With an emphasis on holistic well-being and practical application, the "Chronic Fatigue Syndrome Diet Cookbook" is not just a collection of recipes but a comprehensive guide aimed at improving the quality of life for those managing CFS through thoughtful and informed nutrition. Finally, the cookbook goes beyond the kitchen by guiding on navigating social occasions and dining out with CFS.

CHAPTER ONE

CHRONIC FATIGUE SYNDROME DIET INTRODUCTION

DIETARY INTERVENTIONS FOR CHRONIC FATIGUE SYNDROME

Managing Chronic Fatigue Syndrome (CFS) requires a multimodal approach, with diet playing a critical role in maintaining overall health and effectively managing symptoms. An individually tailored, well-balanced diet can help reduce fatigue, increase energy, and support immune function. Nutritional choices for CFS patients can affect inflammation levels, gut health, and mood stability, all of which are linked to the severity of symptoms. By emphasizing nutrient-dense foods that provide sustained energy without spiking blood sugar, people with CFS can improve their quality of life and manage their condition more effectively.

A diet high in vitamins, minerals, antioxidants, and healthy fats can mitigate oxidative stress and promote cellular function—a crucial aspect for people who suffer from chronic fatigue. Foods high in omega-3 fatty acids, like walnuts, flaxseeds, and fatty fish, can help fight inflammation, and lean proteins, like chicken, turkey, and tofu, provide essential amino acids for immune system support and muscle repair. Complex carbohydrates, found in whole grains and vegetables, offer a consistent energy source while reducing the effects of blood sugar fluctuations that can cause fatigue.

Overall, adopting a balanced and nutritious diet is a cornerstone of managing CFS, promoting resilience, and optimizing daily functioning. People with CFS can stabilize their energy levels throughout the day by focusing on whole, unprocessed foods and avoiding sugary snacks and refined carbohydrates. Hydration is also important, as dehydration can exacerbate fatigue symptoms. Drinking an adequate amount of water and incorporating hydrating foods like fruits and vegetables can support overall energy levels and cognitive function.

With a focus on maximizing nutritional benefits and minimizing triggers that could exacerbate symptoms, the Chronic Fatigue Syndrome Diet Cookbook is a comprehensive resource that offers a variety of nutrient-packed meal ideas that specifically cater to the needs of those managing chronic fatigue. It emphasizes the importance of balanced eating, meaning that every meal supports immune function, energy levels, and overall well-being. The goal of the cookbook is to empower people with CFS to take control of their health through delicious and practical recipes.

Along with recipes, the cookbook offers insightful information on how to choose ingredients, prepare food, and plan meals that are specific to the difficulties faced by people with CFS. Its approach to cooking is straightforward and approachable, making it easier to prepare nourishing meals that support long-term energy and vitality. Whether a person is just getting diagnosed or wants to adjust their diet, this cookbook is a reliable ally on the path to better health and symptom management.

Ultimately, the cookbook aims to improve quality of life by offering doable solutions that support long-term well-being and resilience in managing chronic fatigue. Its main objective is to inspire confidence in the kitchen and encourage a positive relationship with food among individuals with CFS. Through fostering an understanding of how different nutrients can impact symptoms and overall health, the cookbook equips readers with the knowledge needed to make informed dietary choices.

HOW TO MAKE THE MOST OF THIS COOKBOOK

Understanding the Chronic Fatigue Syndrome Diet Cookbook's structure and resources is a good place to start. Go through the introductions to learn about the cookbook's goals, essential dietary guidelines, and advice on how to modify recipes to fit individual tastes and dietary constraints.

All of the recipes are organized into user-friendly categories, like breakfasts, lunches, dinners, and snacks so that you can find meals that fit your preferences and needs quickly.

A wide range of colors and textures should be included when organizing meals because this guarantees a varied spectrum of nutrients. Start by choosing recipes that suit your palate and dietary needs, then gradually try new ingredients to broaden your culinary horizons. The cookbook also promotes creativity in the kitchen by providing ideas for substituting ingredients and advice on how to modify recipes according to seasonal availability or personal preferences.

To get the most out of this resource, utilize the shopping lists and meal planning templates. These tools help people prepare healthy meals more quickly and with less stress. People who plan and cook meals in advance can save time and energy and have nourishing options available to them. They should also regularly consult the cookbook's nutritional guidelines to maintain a balanced diet that promotes optimal health and well-being.

RECOGNIZING CFS NUTRITION FUNDAMENTALS

For people with Chronic Fatigue Syndrome (CFS), eating a diet high in nutrients is essential to maintaining stable energy levels and reducing the severity of symptoms. Deficits in certain essential nutrients, like magnesium, vitamin D, and B12, can worsen fatigue and other symptoms associated with CFS.

Nutrition plays a critical role in managing CFS by providing essential nutrients that support energy production, immune function, and overall well-being.

Foods high in antioxidants, like berries, leafy greens, and nuts, help combat oxidative stress and inflammation, which are common in individuals with CFS. A balanced diet for CFS typically consists of a variety of whole foods such as fruits, vegetables, lean proteins, whole grains, and healthy fats. These foods provide a steady supply of energy and essential nutrients without causing blood sugar spikes, which can contribute to fatigue and mood swings.

Drinking enough water throughout the day supports cellular hydration and helps flush out toxins, promoting overall health and vitality. By prioritizing nutrient-dense foods and staying hydrated, people with CFS can optimize their nutritional intake and support their body's natural ability to heal and recover. Hydration is also essential for managing the symptoms of chronic fatigue syndrome (CFS). Dehydration can exacerbate fatigue and impair cognitive function.

ADVICE ON ORGANIZING AND PREPARING MEALS

For those who are managing Chronic Fatigue Syndrome (CFS), meal preparation and planning are crucial skills because they make it easier to prepare wholesome meals while preserving energy. To start, schedule a specific time each week to plan meals and make a shopping list using the recipes and ingredients found in the cookbook. This proactive approach not only saves time but also makes sure that wholesome options are always available, which lowers the temptation to rely on convenience foods that might be less beneficial to general health.

Batch cooking and meal prepping can be especially helpful for people with CFS, as they enable quick and easy access to pre-prepared meals throughout the week. Select recipes that are easily customizable to individual preferences and dietary restrictions, and experiment with different flavors and ingredients to keep meals interesting and satisfying. A variety of nutrient-dense foods that provide sustained energy and support immune function should be included when planning meals.

To optimize your quality of life and support your health, people with CFS should prioritize convenience. Organize your kitchen and meal prep tools to minimize physical exertion and maximize efficiency. Invest in time-saving kitchen gadgets like an Instant Pot or slow cooker, which can simplify the cooking process while maintaining nutritional integrity.

CHAPTER TWO

COMPREHENDING THE SYNDROME OF CHRONIC FATIGUE

COMPREHENDING THE SYMPTOMS OF CHRONIC FATIGUE SYNDROME

People with Chronic Fatigue Syndrome (CFS), also known as myalgic encephalomyelitis (ME), suffer from a complex and debilitating condition that is characterized by persistent fatigue that does not improve with rest and may worsen with physical or mental activity. The exact cause of CFS is unknown, but it is thought to involve a combination of factors such as immune system dysfunction, viral infections, and hormonal imbalances. People with CFS often experience profound exhaustion that limits their ability to perform daily tasks, affecting both physical and cognitive functions.

Living with CFS can be difficult because symptoms can vary greatly from person to person. Symptoms include sore throat, headaches, muscle and joint pain, extreme fatigue, sleep disturbances, cognitive difficulties (commonly referred to as "brain fog"), and headaches. Diagnosing CFS can be difficult because it involves ruling out other medical conditions that present with similar symptoms through a thorough medical history, physical examination, and occasionally, specialized tests.

SIGNS AND PROGNOSIS

The main symptom of CFS is chronic fatigue that does not go away after six months of no sleep. Other symptoms that are frequently experienced include headaches, unrefreshing sleep, cognitive impairment (such as memory problems or difficulty concentrating), muscle and joint pain, and sore throats. The severity of these symptoms varies from person to person and can be debilitating.

Since there is no specific diagnostic test for CFS, medical professionals must rely on clinical judgment and criteria established by organizations such as the

Centers for Disease Control and Prevention (CDC) and the Institute of Medicine (IOM). To ensure an accurate diagnosis, a comprehensive assessment by a healthcare professional is usually conducted, usually through a process of exclusion wherein other medical conditions with similar symptoms are ruled out.

DIET'S EFFECT ON CFS SYMPTOMS

Dietary changes can help manage symptoms and enhance overall well-being. Many CFS sufferers discover that some foods or dietary practices can exacerbate symptoms like fatigue, digestive problems, and inflammation, while others may provide relief. The importance of diet in managing CFS symptoms is becoming more widely acknowledged.

Reducing refined sugars and processed foods, focusing on whole, nutrient-dense foods, and eliminating potential food sensitivities (like dairy or gluten) are common dietary approaches for managing the symptoms of CFS. Some people may benefit from dicts emphasizing anti-inflammatory foods, like fruits, vegetables, lean proteins, healthy fats (like omega-3 fatty acids), and anti-inflammatory foods. Hydration is also important for managing symptoms like fatigue and cognitive function.

ESSENTIALS OF DIETARY PRACTICES FOR CFS MANAGEMENT

A balanced diet rich in essential nutrients can help regulate energy levels, support immune function, and reduce inflammation. Key nutrients for people with CFS include protein for immune support and muscle repair, healthy fats for brain function and inflammation reduction, and complex carbohydrates for sustained energy. Nutrition plays a pivotal role in managing CFS by supporting overall health and addressing specific symptoms.

Proper timing and portion control can also help stabilize energy levels and prevent digestive discomfort, which are common concerns for those with CFS. Eating a variety of fruits, vegetables, whole grains, and lean proteins can provide essential vitamins and minerals that support overall well-being. Some individuals with CFS may also benefit from supplements under the guidance of a healthcare provider, particularly if deficiencies are identified through blood tests.

Eating regular meals that contain a combination of carbohydrates, proteins, fats, and fiber helps stabilize blood sugar levels and sustain energy throughout the day. This approach can reduce fatigue, improve cognitive function, and support immune system function. Eating balanced meals is essential for individuals with CFS to manage symptoms effectively and support overall health.

A serving of whole grains, such as brown rice or quinoa, a lean protein source, such as tofu or grilled chicken, a variety of colorful, antioxidant-rich vegetables, and a small serving of healthy fats, such as avocado or olive oil, might make up a balanced meal for someone with CFS. Including easy-to-digest foods and avoiding large meals before bedtime can also promote better sleep quality, which is important for people with CFS because they frequently experience sleep disturbances.

People with CFS can optimize their nutrition to better manage their symptoms and enhance their quality of life by emphasizing nutrient-dense foods and mindful eating practices. Speaking with a registered dietitian or other healthcare provider can offer individualized guidance and support in creating a personalized nutrition plan that suits each person's needs and preferences.

CHAPTER THREE

CREATING A CFS-FRIENDLY DIET

ESSENTIAL ELEMENTS FOR HANDLING CFS

It's critical to concentrate on particular nutrients that promote energy production, immunological function, and general well-being to treat Chronic Fatigue Syndrome (CFS) with nutrition. Important nutrients include:

1. Omega-3 Fatty Acids: Essential for addressing symptoms of Chronic exhaustion Syndrome (CFS), such as cognitive impairment and exhaustion, omega-3s are found in fatty fish like salmon, flaxseeds, and walnuts. They also reduce inflammation and improve brain function.

2. Magnesium: Foods high in magnesium, such as whole grains, spinach, and almonds, assist in controlling nerve and muscle function, reducing pain and promoting relaxation. This is advantageous for CFS patients who are feeling stiffness in their muscles.

3. Vitamin D: Sunlight exposure and fortified foods such as cereals and dairy are good sources of this important nutrient, which is also important for immune system function and bone health. Vitamin D deficiency is common among CFS patients.

4. Antioxidants: Included in vibrant fruits and veggies like bell peppers, tomatoes, and berries, antioxidants help to repair cells and support the immune system, which helps with healing and regaining energy. They also fight oxidative stress, which exacerbates the symptoms of chronic fatigue syndrome.

5. B Vitamins: B12 and folate, which are abundant in lean meats, eggs, and leafy greens, are very important for nervous system function and energy production.

ITEMS TO ADD TO YOUR DIET

The main focus of a CFS-friendly diet should be nutrient-dense meals that promote general health and energy levels:

1. Lean Proteins: Include foods such as fish, chicken, beans, and tofu. These sources include vital amino acids needed for energy production and muscle repair.

2. Complex Carbohydrates: To counteract weariness and stabilize mood, choose whole grains like quinoa, brown rice, and oats, which offer continuous energy without spiking blood sugar levels.

3. Healthy Fats: Consume foods high in omega-3 fatty acids, such as avocados, almonds, and olive oil, as these enhance general health and cognitive performance.

4. Vibrant Fruits and Vegetables: Choose a range of colors to guarantee a wide range of antioxidants, vitamins, and minerals that boost immunity and reduce inflammation.

5. Hydration: Staying hydrated is essential for controlling CFS symptoms. Drink lots of water throughout the day to sustain overall body functions and energy levels.

It's critical to limit foods that can worsen symptoms or cause inflammation to effectively treat CFS:

1. Processed meals: Steer clear of meals that are heavy in additives, preservatives, and refined sugars as these ingredients can exacerbate weariness and cause energy dips.

2. Limit your intake of alcohol and caffeine: These substances can cause sleep disturbances and make exhaustion and dehydration worse, which are common problems for people with CFS.

3. High-Sodium Foods: Limit your intake of processed meats, canned goods, and salty snacks since these can increase fluid retention and make symptoms like fatigue and bloating worse.

4. Gluten and Dairy: Since gluten and dairy can aggravate inflammation and digestive problems, some people with CFS find relief from cutting back on or avoiding them.

Identifying triggers can be achieved by experimenting with elimination diets under physician supervision.

5. Artificial Sweeteners: Steer clear of artificial sweeteners as they may aggravate symptoms like weariness and upset stomach by interfering with gut health and metabolism.

SAMPLE MENUS FOR VARIOUS LIFESTYLES

Developing well-rounded meal plans that accommodate various lifestyles can aid in the efficient management of CFS symptoms:

1. Busy Professional

• Oatmeal made the night before with chia seeds and berries on top.

• Lunch consists of grilled chicken salad topped with avocado, mixed greens, and vinaigrette dressing.

• Supper consists of quinoa, roasted veggies, and baked salmon.

2. Vegan or Vegetarian:

• Smoothie made with protein powder, banana, spinach, and almond milk for breakfast.

• Lentil and vegetable stew served with whole grain toast for lunch.

• Steamed broccoli and brown rice paired with stir-fried tofu for dinner.

3. Athlete or Intense Person:

• Whole grain bread with sliced banana and almond butter for breakfast.

• Turkey wrap with whole grain tortilla, hummus, and spinach for lunch.

• Supper is grilled lean steak over sautéed greens and sweet potatoes.

MODIFYING DIET DEPENDING ON SYMPTOMS

Adaptability in diet modification in response to symptoms is essential for successful CFS management:

1. Fatigue: To sustain energy levels throughout the day, concentrate on consuming simple-to-digest foods like soups, smoothies, and short, frequent meals.

2. Muscular Pain: To promote muscular relaxation and repair, raise your consumption of meals high in magnesium and lean proteins.

3. Cognitive Problems: To enhance brain function and clarity, give priority to foods high in omega-3s and antioxidants.

4. Digestive Problems: Under physician supervision, try a low-FODMAP or elimination diet to find trigger foods that can make you feel more uncomfortable in your stomach.

5. Sleep Disturbances: To promote healthy sleep, limit caffeine and alcohol consumption shortly before bed, and include meals high in tryptophan, such as turkey or seeds.

Through the integration of various dietary techniques and customization to specific requirements and symptoms, people suffering from CFS can enhance their overall quality of life and effectively manage their disease.

CHAPTER FOUR

COOKING METHODS AND ADVICE

HEALTHY COOKING TECHNIQUES

Cooking healthy meals for people with Chronic Fatigue Syndrome (CFS) requires careful consideration of which cooking techniques to use. For example, using steaming, baking, or grilling instead of frying helps cut down on unhealthy fat intake; steaming vegetables retain their vitamins and minerals better than boiling, which can strip them of their nutrients; baking or roasting meats and fish without added oils can preserve their natural flavors while keeping them tender and juicy; and grilling adds a delicious smoky taste without going overboard in fat.

A healthy cooking technique that is also beneficial is stir-frying vegetables in a small amount of oil over high heat; this method cooks them quickly without sacrificing their crunch or nutritional value. Moreover, you can use a variety of vegetables, which improves the dish's flavor profile and nutrient density. Using non-stick cookware also helps you control fat intake by using less oil, so you can make tasty meals that are satisfying and enjoyable for people with CFS.

ADVICE FOR MAINTAINING NUTRITION IN FOODS

Meal preservation is important for people with Chronic Fatigue Syndrome because it can support overall health and energy levels. To start, use fresh, high-quality ingredients because they usually contain more nutrients than processed ones. When boiling or steaming fruits and vegetables, use as little water as possible to preserve water-soluble vitamins like vitamin C and B-complex vitamins. Cooking vegetables until they are just tender helps retain their nutrients, so they stay flavorful and full of vital vitamins and minerals.

Meats and fish should not be overcooked; instead, cooking techniques that retain moisture and nutrients, like steaming or poaching, should be used; soaking grains and legumes before cooking can improve nutrient absorption and shorten cooking times; adding a range of vibrant fruits and vegetables to meals adds color and appeal while guaranteeing a varied intake of vitamins, minerals, and antioxidants; with these suggestions, you can optimize meal nutritional value and meet the dietary requirements of people with CFS.

TIME-SAVING TECHNIQUES FOR PREPARING MEALS

For people with Chronic Fatigue Syndrome, meal preparation efficiency is critical because it reduces energy use and guarantees a steady supply of nutrient-dense meals. To start, plan meals ahead of time and make a weekly meal plan to make grocery shopping and preparation easier. Make use of batch cooking methods by making large amounts of staple foods like grains, proteins, and sauces that can be portioned and frozen for easy assembly throughout the week. Investing in time-saving kitchen appliances like a pressure cooker or slow cookers can speed up cooking times while adding flavor to food.

Make easy-to-eat snacks and meals that only need to be partially assembled, like pre-cut veggies with hummus or yogurt parfaits with fresh fruit and nuts. Make inventive use of leftover ingredients by repurposing them in other meals or creating new dishes to cut down on food waste and save time. Choose straightforward recipes that call for fewer ingredients and shorter cooking times without sacrificing taste or nutrition. By implementing these time-saving techniques, you can simplify meal preparation for people with CFS and make it simpler for them to maintain a balanced diet without experiencing undue stress or exhaustion.

RECIPES FOR SIMPLE AND FAST DINNERS

Meal planning is crucial for people with Chronic Fatigue Syndrome because it guarantees that they will eat a healthy diet without burning too much energy. One-pot meals, such as thick soups or stews full of vegetables and lean proteins, are easy to make and offer a full meal in a bowl. Stir-fries made with cooked grains or proteins and pre-cut vegetables can be put together quickly and flavored with sauces or seasonings. Salads with a range of fresh ingredients, such as leafy greens, nuts, seeds, and lean proteins, are not only easy to put together but also nutrient-dense and filling.

Smoothies made with fruits, vegetables, yogurt, and protein powder are a great way to get all the nutrients you need in one serving for breakfast or a snack. You can make overnight oats the night before with rolled oats, milk or yogurt, and toppings like fresh fruit or nuts for a hassle-free breakfast option. You can also use ingredients like canned beans, canned fish, or frozen vegetables to make recipes more time-efficient while still maintaining a balanced meal.

COOKING TO MEET A VARIETY OF DIETARY REQUIREMENTS

Various dietary restrictions must be accommodated when cooking for people with Chronic Fatigue Syndrome, so creativity and careful ingredient selection are key. First, become familiar with common dietary restrictions, such as lactose intolerance, gluten intolerance, and allergies to particular foods, like shellfish or nuts.

Plan meals that are easily modified or customized to meet these restrictions, like providing dairy-free or gluten-free options for sauces and desserts. You can also use alternative ingredients, like almond flour, coconut milk, or nutritional yeast, to replace traditional allergens without sacrificing taste or texture.

Dishes should be labeled with ingredients and potential allergens to help people with CFS make educated food choices. When cooking for others, try making a variety of dishes that accommodate varying dietary preferences and restrictions to make sure everyone is included and has fun. Try trying out international cuisines that naturally fit into certain dietary restrictions, like Mediterranean or vegetarian dishes that focus on fresh produce, legumes, and healthy fats. By embracing a variety of ingredients and culinary techniques, you can make tasty and filling meals that effectively meet the dietary requirements of people with CFS.

CHAPTER FIVE

MEAL PLANNING: RECIPES FOR BREAKFAST

HEALTHY SHAKES AND SMOOTHIES

Smoothies and shakes made with healthy ingredients are easy to make and a great way to get your nutrients and energy up in the morning. Begin by choosing a range of frozen or fresh fruits, like mangoes, bananas, or berries, which add sweetness vitamins, and antioxidants. To make the smoothie even more nutritious, add some leafy greens, like kale or spinach, which are high in fiber and micronutrients.

If you want your smoothie to be extra creamy, add a base such as Greek yogurt, almond milk, or soy milk. These will add protein and healthy fats. You can also add extras like chia seeds for omega-3s, oats for long-lasting energy, or a scoop of protein powder for muscle recovery. Blend until smooth and transfer into a glass or travel container for a wholesome breakfast that will keep you full all morning.

Discover your favorite smoothie blend by experimenting with different flavor combinations and ingredient ratios. Whether you're craving a green smoothie loaded with vegetables or a tropical fruit medley, the possibilities are endless. When you become an expert smoothie maker, you'll wake up feeling energized and prepared to take on the day.

BREAKFAST BOWLS THAT INVIGORATE

Breakfast bowls are a versatile and aesthetically pleasing way to pack a nutritional punch into your morning meal. Start with a healthy base, like quinoa, overnight oats, or Greek yogurt, which are all high in fiber and protein. Then, top your bowl with colorful fresh fruit, like sliced strawberries, blueberries, or kiwis, which add natural sweetness and vital vitamins.

To enhance the texture and taste, mix in nuts and seeds (almonds, chia seeds, or pumpkin seeds), which add crunch and healthy fats; drizzle with nut butter or honey for additional sweetness and richness; or add superfoods (goji berries, cacao nibs, or hemp hearts), which each have their special health benefits.

Power breakfast bowls are adaptable to accommodate a wide range of dietary requirements and palates, which makes them a great option for anyone looking for a filling and healthy breakfast. When you mix healthful ingredients with eye-catching toppings, you can make a breakfast bowl that will not only satisfy your hunger but also awaken your senses and make your day.

OPTIONS FOR HIGH-PROTEIN BREAKFASTS

Lean meats like turkey or chicken sausage, eggs, or plant-based substitutes like tempeh or tofu are high in protein and provide the essential amino acids needed for muscle growth and repair. A high-protein breakfast is crucial for maintaining energy levels and accelerating muscle recovery throughout the day.

Add leafy greens or vegetables like spinach, tomatoes, or peppers to boost nutrient density and add color to your plate.

For a balanced meal, include healthy fats from sources like avocado, nuts, or olive oil, which promote satiety and support overall health. Pair your protein source with complex carbohydrates like whole-grain toast, sweet potatoes, or oatmeal, which provide sustained energy and fiber.

Try different ways to cook, like baking a frittata for an easy make-ahead option or scrambling eggs with veggies. When you prioritize protein for breakfast, you can properly fuel your body and establish a good example for the rest of the day, which will ensure that you have energy and perform at your best.

IDEAS FOR QUICK BREAKFASTS

Convenient yet nutritious, grab-and-go breakfast ideas are ideal for hectic mornings. To make them, make overnight oats or chia seed pudding the night before, letting the ingredients soak and flavor each other. You can personalize these portable options by adding nuts, seeds, or fresh fruits as toppings, which will provide a healthy balance of carbohydrates, protein, and healthy fats.

For a savory twist, try making mini quiches or egg muffins loaded with cheese and vegetables, which can be eaten cold or quickly reheated. Another quick option is a whole-grain breakfast bar or muffin, made ahead of time and stored for easy access. Opt for recipes that include ingredients like oats, whole-wheat flour, and dried fruits, which provide sustained energy and natural sweetness.

Smoothies that are travel-friendly or a homemade trail mix that includes nuts, seeds, and dried fruits are also great options for on-the-go breakfasts. These ideas guarantee that you get a healthy start to the day, even if you're pressed for time, and will help you stay focused and full until your next meal.

RECIPES FOR GRANOLA AND BARS MADE AT HOME

Making your granola and bars gives you complete control over what goes into them and the flavors you like, making them a healthy and filling breakfast option. To start, combine rolled oats, nuts, seeds, and dried fruits in a large mixing bowl and toss with a mixture of honey or maple syrup and a small pinch of vanilla extract. Spread the mixture evenly on a baking sheet and bake, stirring occasionally to ensure even toasting, until golden brown.

For homemade bars, combine oats with nut butter, honey, and optional ingredients like chocolate chips or coconut flakes. Press the mixture into a lined baking dish, refrigerate until set, and then cut into bars for an easy grab-and-go breakfast or snack. Once cooled, break the granola into clusters and store it in an airtight container for up to two weeks. Enjoy it with yogurt or milk for a crunchy breakfast treat.

Learn how to customize your granola and bars to your taste preferences and dietary requirements by experimenting with different flavor combinations and ingredients such as protein powder, dried berries, and cinnamon.

By perfecting these homemade recipes, you can make sure your breakfast is not only delicious but also full of healthy ingredients to start your day.

Whether you prefer a quick grab-and-go option or enjoy taking the time to prepare a wholesome breakfast bowl or smoothie, these breakfast ideas offer a range of options to suit different tastes and dietary preferences, ensuring you can start your day with a nutritious and satisfying meal. Including these recipes in your morning routine can help you maintain energy levels, support overall health, and set a positive tone for the day ahead.

FRESH SALADS AND DRESSINGS

A staple of any Chronic Fatigue Syndrome (CFS) diet, fresh salads give you those necessary nutrients without making you feel heavy. Begin with a base of colorful greens like spinach or kale, then add a variety of colorful vegetables for crunch and flavor, such as bell peppers, cherry tomatoes, and cucumber slices; for added protein, add lean sources like grilled chicken breast or chickpeas; and for texture and healthy fats, add nuts or seeds like almonds or sunflower seeds.

Make your dressings to keep ingredients under control and steer clear of additives. Basic vinaigrette made with olive oil, balsamic vinegar, Dijon mustard, and a dash of honey or maple syrup will go well with your salad; try different herbs, like cilantro or basil, for a novel twist. It's all about striking a balance between flavors and wholesome, nourishing ingredients.

Sauté aromatics like onions, garlic, and celery in olive oil until fragrant, then add hearty vegetables like carrots, sweet potatoes, and spinach, along with protein sources like beans or lentils for sustained energy. Soups and stews are comforting and ideal for CFS because they provide warmth and plenty of nutrients in one bowl.

A complete and satisfying meal that supports your health and energy levels throughout the day can be made by adding anti-inflammatory herbs and spices like thyme, rosemary, turmeric, and ginger to enhance flavors. To reduce salt intake, use low-sodium broth or homemade stock. Simmer everything together until the vegetables are tender and the flavors meld beautifully. Serve hot with a slice of whole-grain bread.

IDEAS FOR A NOURISHING SANDWICH AND WRAP

For a CFS-friendly lunch, sandwiches, and wraps can be a wholesome and portable option. To start, use whole-grain bread or wraps as a base, as they offer complex carbohydrates for sustained energy and can be filled with lean proteins like turkey, grilled chicken, or tofu for muscle repair and satiety.

For extra flavor and creaminess, spread hummus, guacamole, or a homemade yogurt-based dressing instead of high-fat condiments; roll them up or cut them into halves for easy handling, and enjoy a balanced meal that's simple to pack for on-the-go lunches. Add plenty of fresh vegetables, such as lettuce, sliced tomatoes, avocado, and shredded carrots, for fiber and vitamins.

Adding a variety of colorful vegetables, like roasted sweet potatoes, steamed broccoli, and raw bell peppers for vitamins and minerals, to a base of whole grains, like quinoa, brown rice, or couscous, provides complex carbohydrates and fiber. Healthy lunch bowls: With CFS, lunch bowls are versatile and allow for endless combinations to suit your taste and dietary needs.

Add lean proteins (grilled salmon, chickpeas, or diced tofu) to help with energy and muscle repair. Garnish with a homemade dressing or sauce (made from natural ingredients like tahini, lemon juice, and herbs) for extra flavor without added sugar or sodium. Blend everything thoroughly or divide the ingredients into sections for a visually appealing and filling lunch bowl.

Make your energy bars with oats, almonds, seeds, and dried fruit for a balanced snack. Portable snacks are great for controlling your CFS symptoms during the day. Choose snacks that combine protein and fiber for long-lasting energy.

Fresh fruit with almonds or a small bowl of Greek yogurt with honey and berries are other great options. Snacking on raw veggies like carrots and celery dipped in hummus or guacamole is also a great way to get your nutrients in quickly. Make these snacks ahead of time and store them in portioned containers or resealable bags so you can easily grab them anytime you get hungry.

HEALTHY ONE-POT DINNERS

Incorporating all ingredients into a single pot allows flavors to meld together beautifully. Whether it's chicken, beef, or plant-based options like tofu or beans, sauté your protein with aromatics like onions and garlic until browned and fragrant. Next, add in vegetables of your choice—think bell peppers, carrots, and zucchini—for added nutrients and texture. Healthy one-pot meals are a lifesaver for busy evenings or when you simply want to minimize cleanup while maximizing flavor.

After the protein and veggies are cooked to perfection, add your grains or starches—rice, quinoa, or pasta—along with broth or water to cook them thoroughly. Season liberally with herbs and spices, like paprika, cumin, rosemary, or thyme, to enhance the flavor. Simmer everything together until the grains are soft and have absorbed the flavors of the dish. Garnish with chopped fresh herbs, like cilantro or parsley, for a burst of freshness, and serve immediately from the pot. One-pot meals are easy to prepare and guarantee a delicious and filling supper without the trouble of having to clean up multiple dishes afterward.

Cozy casseroles and bakes are ideal for lazy Sundays or entertaining because they simply require layering ingredients in a baking dish and leaving it to bake. Pick your base—pasta, potatoes, or grains like quinoa—cook it until it's fork-tender, then layer it in the baking dish with your protein of choice—ground meat, chicken, or lentils for a vegetarian option—and top it off with lots of veggies—spices, broccoli, or mushrooms for extra flavor and nutrition.

To bind everything together, make a creamy or cheesy sauce (you can use a basic béchamel sauce made with butter, flour, and milk, or you can use vegetable broth and nutritional yeast for a vegan option). Pour the sauce over your layered ingredients, making sure to coat everything well. Garnish your casserole with cheese, breadcrumbs, or a sprinkle of herbs for a crispy, golden finish. Bake in the oven until bubbling and the top is golden brown.

Allow it to rest for a few minutes before serving. Casseroles and bakes are comforting and adaptable—you can adjust the ingredients to suit your diet or what's in season.

TASTY STIR-FRIES AND SKILLET DINNERS

Quick cooking and bright flavors are the keys to flavorful stir-fries and skillet meals that come together quickly and are ideal for busy weeknights. Heat some oil in a skillet or wok over medium-high heat, then add your protein (be it thinly sliced beef, chicken strips, or tofu) and cook until it's browned and cooked through. Take the protein out of the skillet and set it aside.

Add your favorite veggies (broccoli, bell peppers, and snap peas are great options) to the skillet and stir-fry until the veggies are crisp-tender. Then, return the cooked protein to the skillet and add your sauce (you can use a tomato-based sauce for a Mediterranean touch or a simple soy sauce, garlic, and ginger mixture for an Asian flavor). Toss everything together until well combined and heated through.

Serve your stir-fry over cooked rice, noodles, or quinoa for a complete meal. For extra texture and freshness, top with chopped green onions, sesame seeds, or fresh herbs. Stir-fries and skillet meals are delicious and adaptable, letting you make a filling supper quickly out of leftover veggies and proteins.

Vegetarian and vegan dinner options are vibrant, flavorful, and satisfying, showcasing the versatility of plant-based ingredients. Start by choosing your protein substitute—whether it's tofu, tempeh, lentils, or beans—that will form the heart of your dish. Prepare your protein substitute by marinating it in herbs, spices, or a flavorful sauce to enhance its taste.

Next, select a variety of colorful vegetables to add texture and nutrition. Think of bell peppers, eggplant, spinach, and mushrooms, each bringing its unique flavor profile to the dish. Sauté your vegetables in a skillet or wok with a drizzle of olive oil until tender and slightly caramelized.

Combine your prepared protein substitute and vegetables in the skillet, stirring gently to mix everything. Add a sauce or seasoning of your choice—whether it's a creamy coconut curry, a zesty lemon herb dressing, or a spicy peanut sauce—to tie all the tastes together.

Serve your vegetarian or vegan creation over cooked grains like quinoa or brown rice, or enjoy it as a standalone dish. Garnish with fresh herbs, toasted nuts, or a drizzle of olive oil for added flavor and visual appeal. Vegetarian and vegan dinner options are not only nutritious but also delicious, showcasing the abundance of plant-based ingredients available for creating satisfying meals.

Recipes for slow cooker and Instant Pot dishes are perfect for those who prefer a hands-off approach to cooking without compromising on flavor. These appliances are ideal for tenderizing meats, simmering stews, and infusing flavors over long periods.

For slow cooker dishes, start by layering your ingredients directly into the slow cooker inserts. Choose your protein—such as beef, chicken, or pork—and place it at the bottom for even cooking. Add root vegetables like carrots, potatoes, and onions around the protein, ensuring they will cook evenly and absorb the flavors.

Pour in your chosen liquid—whether it's broth, wine, or a flavorful sauce—to keep everything moist during the slow cooking process. Season generously with herbs and spices like bay leaves, thyme, or paprika for added depth of flavor.

Cover the slow cooker with its lid and set it to cook on low for several hours, allowing the ingredients to meld together and become tender. Once cooked, garnish with fresh herbs or a squeeze of lemon juice before serving.

For Instant Pot recipes, start by sautéing your aromatics—such as onions, garlic, and ginger—in the Instant Pot using the sauté option. Add your protein and sear it until browned on all sides to improve its taste.

Next, add your vegetables, grains, and liquid—such as broth or water—to the Instant Pot, ensuring everything is thoroughly blended. Close the lid and set the Instant Pot to pressure cook for the stated time according to your recipe.

Once the cooking cycle is complete, let the pressure relax normally or do a rapid release, depending on the recipe's requirements. Stir everything together gently and adjust the seasoning if needed before serving.

Both slow cooker and Instant Pot dishes are convenient and versatile, allowing you to prepare delicious meals with minimal effort and maximum flavor.

NUTRITIOUS SNACK RECIPES

Discovering nutritious snack recipes is key to maintaining energy levels throughout the day while managing chronic fatigue syndrome. These snacks should ideally combine protein, healthy fats, and complex carbohydrates for sustained energy. Consider recipes like hummus with veggie sticks, Greek yogurt with berries and nuts, or homemade trail mix with seeds and dried fruits. These options are easy to prepare and can be stored for quick access during fatigue episodes. By focusing on nutrient-dense ingredients, these snacks not only provide energy but also support overall health and well-being.

HEALTHY DESSERT ALTERNATIVES

Finding healthy dessert alternatives that satisfy sweet cravings without compromising health is essential for that managing chronic fatigue syndrome. Opt for desserts made with natural sweeteners like honey or maple syrup instead of refined sugars. Recipes such as fruit sorbets made from blended frozen fruits, chia seed puddings with almond milk, or baked apples with cinnamon offer delicious options with lower sugar content. These desserts are not only nutritious but also rich in vitamins, minerals, and antioxidants, promoting better immune function and overall energy levels.

ENERGY-BOOSTING SMOOTHIE BOWLS

Energy-boosting smoothie bowls are perfect for breakfast or as a snack to combat fatigue and maintain nutrition. Blend ingredients like leafy greens, fruits, nut butter, and protein-rich additions such as Greek yogurt or tofu. Top with superfoods like chia seeds, hemp seeds, or granola for added texture and nutrients. Smoothie bowls are customizable, allowing individuals to tailor them to their taste preferences and nutritional needs. They provide a refreshing way to boost energy levels while ensuring the intake of essential vitamins and minerals crucial for managing chronic fatigue syndrome effectively.

Indulging in guilt-free sweet treats is possible with recipes that focus on wholesome ingredients and minimal added sugars. Consider options like avocado chocolate mousse sweetened with dates, banana oat cookies made with whole grain oats and mashed bananas, or coconut macaroons using unsweetened shredded coconut and egg whites. These treats are satisfying yet nutritious, offering a balance of carbohydrates and healthy fats. By choosing these alternatives, individuals can enjoy desserts without worrying about energy crashes or exacerbating symptoms of chronic fatigue syndrome.

RECIPES FOR HOMEMADE ENERGY BARS

Creating homemade energy bars ensures control over ingredients and customization based on personal dietary needs. Use a base of oats, nuts, and seeds combined with binding agents like honey or nut butter. Add-ins such as dried fruits, cocoa nibs, or spices like cinnamon can enhance flavor and nutritional value. These bars are convenient for quick energy boosts and can be prepared in batches for easy storage. Homemade energy bars provide sustained energy release, making them ideal for managing fatigue while providing essential nutrients crucial for overall health and well-being.

RECIPES FOR HYDRATING DRINKS

Maintaining optimal hydration levels throughout the day is imperative for managing chronic fatigue syndrome (CFS). To start your day off right, make a refreshing cucumber mint water by simply adding cucumber slices and fresh mint leaves to a pitcher of water and letting it infuse overnight in the refrigerator. This drink is not only delicious but also aids in detoxifying the body and keeps you hydrated.

Another fantastic way to stay hydrated is to combine coconut water with a little pineapple juice. Pineapple juice adds flavor and vitamin C, which boosts energy and the immune system. Coconut water is naturally high in electrolytes, so it's a great way to replace minerals lost from exhaustion or dehydration.

Try making a batch of hibiscus iced tea for a hydrating take on traditional tea. Packed with antioxidants that support cardiovascular health and fight inflammation, hibiscus tea is known for its refreshing tart flavor; you can sweeten it with a little honey or agave syrup for a guilt-free hydrating treat that you can enjoy all day.

Herbal teas are a great way to naturally reduce stress and increase energy levels, which makes them ideal for managing the symptoms of chronic fatigue syndrome. For a calming and restorative cup of tea at bedtime, steep dried chamomile flowers in hot water for a few minutes, strain, and enjoy with a drizzle of honey.

Another herbal remedy that can stimulate the senses and improve mental clarity is peppermint tea. Its cooling qualities can help reduce headaches and ease digestive discomfort, which are common symptoms of chronic fatigue syndrome. To use peppermint tea, steep dried or fresh peppermint leaves in boiling water for five to ten minutes, then slowly sip.

A pot of ginseng tea can help you feel more energized naturally. It has been used for centuries in traditional medicine because of its adaptogenic qualities, which help the body handle stress and improve stamina. You can enjoy it as a mid-afternoon pick-me-up by adding a slice of lemon or a little honey to balance the slightly bitter taste.

BLENDS OF FRESH JUICE FOR NUTRITION

A revitalizing green juice blend can include kale, spinach, cucumber, celery, and a splash of lemon juice. Green vegetables are rich in antioxidants and chlorophyll, which help cleanse the body and naturally boost energy levels. Fresh juices are packed with vitamins, minerals, and antioxidants that can support overall health and combat fatigue.

Try a vibrant carrot-orange-ginger juice for a sweeter option. The combination of carrots' high beta-carotene content and the high vitamin C content of oranges, along with the added benefit of ginger's digestive aids, makes this juice blend both nutrient-dense and easy on the stomach.

SMOOTHIES AS A RAPID SOURCE OF NUTRIENTS

A classic banana-berry smoothie contains bananas, mixed berries, Greek yogurt, and a splash of almond milk. Rich in potassium, which supports muscle function and electrolyte balance, berries offer antioxidants that combat oxidative stress. Smoothies are convenient and nutrient-dense, making them an ideal choice for busy days when you need a quick energy boost.

Blend spinach, avocado, almond butter, and a scoop of protein powder for a high-protein smoothie option. Spinach is a great source of iron, which is important for preventing fatigue, avocado adds creaminess and healthy fats, almond butter and protein powder support muscle recovery, and protein powder gives you sustained energy.

RECIPES FOR DRINKS THAT CALM THE NIGHT

Comforting beverages for bedtime can help with chronic fatigue syndrome management by fostering relaxation and improving the quality of sleep. One such beverage is a warm golden milk latte, which is made with turmeric, cinnamon, ginger, and coconut milk. Turmeric has anti-inflammatory properties due to its content of curcumin, and ginger helps with digestion and eases soreness in the muscles.

Alternatively, a cup of warm herbal lavender tea can help calm the mind and prepare the body for sleep. Lavender is revered for its relaxing effects and can reduce anxiety, making it an excellent choice for winding down before bedtime. Steep dried lavender buds in hot water for 5-7 minutes, then strain and enjoy with a touch of honey if desired.

These soothing drinks for bedtime not only help you relax but also support your overall health and well-being. Restful sleep is essential for effectively managing the symptoms of chronic fatigue syndrome, so include these drinks in your daily routine to create a calming atmosphere and enhance the quality of your sleep naturally.

CHAPTER SIX

SPECIAL CONSIDERATIONS

MANAGING DIETARY RESTRICTIONS

For people with Chronic Fatigue Syndrome (CFS), controlling dietary restrictions like gluten-free and dairy-free diets is critical to reducing symptoms and enhancing overall health. Gluten-free diets avoid grains like wheat, barley, and rye, which can aggravate inflammation and digestive problems in some CFS sufferers.

Dairy-free diets avoid dairy products, which can cause discomfort or inflammation in the digestive tract. To successfully control these dietary restrictions, one must emphasize whole foods like fruits, vegetables, lean proteins, and gluten-free grains like quinoa or rice. By incorporating nutrient-dense foods, one can guarantee adequate intake of vital vitamins and minerals, supporting overall health and symptom management.

Gluten-free flour blends and plant-based milk substitutes (such as using almond milk instead of cow's milk in recipes) can help mitigate the digestive problems associated with dairy consumption. Experimenting with different gluten-free grains, such as buckwheat or millet, expands dietary variety while meeting individual preferences and needs. Carefully reading food labels can also help identify hidden gluten or dairy ingredients in packaged foods. Individuals with CFS can maintain a balanced diet that supports their health and well-being by focusing on nutrient-rich, naturally gluten-free, and dairy-free foods.

RECIPES FOR HANDLING TYPICAL SYMPTOMS OF CFS

Recipes that are adapted to address common symptoms of CFS, like inflammation and digestive problems, can greatly enhance quality of life. To support gut health and regular bowel movements, include foods high in fiber, such as fruits, vegetables, and legumes. Ginger, peppermint, or chamomile can be used in recipes to ease the discomfort that comes with digestive problems that many CFS sufferers experience. Recipes that are high in omega-3 fatty acids, which can be found in fish like salmon or flaxseeds, can help reduce inflammation and joint pain that is linked to CFS. Turmeric, when added to recipes, provides a natural anti-inflammatory boost, supporting overall symptom management.

Eating meals that emphasize whole, unprocessed foods guarantees that the intake of nutrients is optimal to support energy levels and general health. Easy recipes such as grilled chicken salads with avocado or vegetable stir-fries with quinoa offer balanced nutrition and are quick and nutritious for those who are managing fatigue. Herbs and spices such as garlic, basil, and cilantro enhance flavor without adding extra salt or unhealthy fats, making meals tasty and helpful for managing CFS symptoms.

ADJUSTING RECIPES FOR WEIGHT MANAGEMENT

Adjusting recipes for weight management is essential for individuals with CFS, as maintaining a healthy weight can support overall well-being and symptom management. Choosing recipes that emphasize lean proteins such as chicken, fish, or tofu helps build muscle mass and promote satiety, reducing the risk of weight fluctuations common in CFS. Incorporating high-fiber foods like whole grains, beans, and vegetables into recipes supports digestive health and helps regulate appetite, contributing to weight management goals. Avoiding refined sugars and processed foods in recipes reduces empty calories and supports stable energy levels throughout the day.

Balancing macronutrients like carbohydrates, proteins, and healthy fats in recipes ensures comprehensive nutrition while supporting weight management efforts. Recipes that include complex carbohydrates such as sweet potatoes or quinoa provide sustained energy without spiking blood sugar levels, promoting stable energy throughout the day. Incorporating healthy fats like avocado, nuts, or olive oil adds flavor and satiety to meals while supporting heart health and overall well-being. Adjusting portion sizes to align with individual energy needs and activity levels further supports weight management goals. By focusing on nutrient-dense, balanced recipes, individuals with CFS can achieve and maintain a healthy weight while supporting their overall health.

NUTRITIONAL SUPPLEMENTS AND THEIR ROLE

Nutritional supplements play a crucial role in supporting the health and well-being of individuals with Chronic Fatigue Syndrome (CFS) by addressing nutrient deficiencies and supporting overall energy levels.

Supplements such as vitamin D3 can help regulate immune function and improve mood, which are commonly affected in individuals with CFS. Omega-3 fatty acids supplements derived from fish oil or algae oil provide anti-inflammatory benefits and support heart health, which is important for individuals managing inflammation associated with CFS. Coenzyme Q10 supplements can enhance cellular energy production, potentially alleviating fatigue symptoms and improving ovcrall energy levels.

Incorporating supplements like magnesium or B vitamins support nervous system function and energy metabolism, addressing common deficiencies observed in individuals with CFS. Consulting with a healthcare provider or registered dietitian helps determine appropriate supplement dosages based on individual needs and health status. It's essential to choose high-quality supplements from reputable brands to ensure purity and efficacy. Integrating supplements into a comprehensive treatment plan that includes a balanced diet and lifestyle modifications optimizes health outcomes for individuals with CFS. By addressing nutrient deficiencies and supporting overall health with targeted supplements, individuals can effectively manage symptoms and improve their quality of life.

DINING OUT AND SOCIAL OCCASIONS WITH CFS

Navigating dining out and social occasions can be challenging for individuals with Chronic Fatigue Syndrome (CFS), but with thoughtful planning and preparation, it's possible to enjoy these experiences while managing symptoms effectively. Choosing restaurants that offer diverse menu options, including gluten-free or dairy-free choices, allows individuals with CFS to adhere to their dietary preferences and restrictions. Communicating dietary needs with restaurant staff helps ensure meals are prepared according to individual requirements, minimizing the risk of digestive discomfort or allergic reactions.

Opting for grilled, steamed, or roasted dishes over fried or heavily processed foods supports overall health and symptom management.

Preparing for social occasions by eating a small, balanced meal or snack beforehand helps regulate blood sugar levels and reduces the temptation to indulge in unhealthy foods. Bringing portable snacks like nuts, seeds, or fruit can provide a nutritious option if suitable food choices are limited. Choosing beverages like herbal tea, sparkling water, or freshly squeezed juices without added sugars supports hydration and overall well-being during social gatherings.

Balancing food intake with rest breaks and pacing activities helps manage fatigue levels and enhances the enjoyment of social interactions. By prioritizing dietary needs and making informed choices, individuals with CFS can participate in dining out and social occasions while supporting their health and well-being.

CHAPTER SEVEN

ADDRESSING FATIGUE-RELATED CHALLENGES IN COOKING

Living with chronic fatigue syndrome (CFS) can present unique challenges, especially when it comes to cooking. Fatigue often makes even simple tasks feel overwhelming. To manage this, it's crucial to simplify meal preparation. Choose recipes that require minimal chopping and cooking time. Opt for slow cookers or one-pot meals that allow you to combine ingredients easily. Preparing large batches and freezing portions can also save energy on days when cooking feels daunting.

Additionally, organizing your kitchen for efficiency can make a significant difference. Keep frequently used utensils and ingredients within easy reach. Use lightweight cookware and ergonomic tools to reduce strain. Planning meals and creating a shopping list based on easy-to-prepare, nutritious foods can streamline the cooking process. Embracing shortcuts like pre-cut vegetables or frozen ingredients can further ease fatigue-related challenges.

Lastly, prioritize self-care and pacing yourself. Take breaks as needed during meal preparation. Consider asking for help from family or using meal delivery services on particularly fatigued days. By adapting your cooking routine and environment, you can manage fatigue more effectively while still enjoying nutritious meals.

HOW TO MAINTAIN A BALANCED DIET DURING FLARE-UPS

During flare-ups of chronic fatigue syndrome (CFS), maintaining a balanced diet is crucial for managing symptoms and supporting overall health. Focus on nutrient-dense foods that provide sustained energy. Include plenty of fruits, vegetables, lean proteins, and whole grains in your diet. Consider small, frequent meals to avoid energy crashes. Plan meals that are easy to digest and gentle on the stomach.

Hydration is also essential. Drink plenty of water throughout the day to support hydration and energy levels. Avoid excessive caffeine and sugary drinks, as they can lead to energy fluctuations. Incorporate healthy fats like avocados, nuts, and olive oil into your meals to help maintain satiety and provide essential nutrients.

When experiencing severe fatigue, consider simpler meal options such as smoothies, soups, or salads. These can be prepared quickly and require minimal energy expenditure. Use herbs and spices to enhance flavors without relying on excessive salt or sugar. By focusing on nutrient-rich foods and adjusting your diet during flare-ups, you can support your body's needs while managing the challenges of chronic fatigue syndrome.

TIPS FOR GROCERY SHOPPING AND MEAL PREPARATION ON LOW-ENERGY DAYS

Meal preparation and grocery shopping can be difficult chores on low-energy days brought on by chronic fatigue syndrome (CFS).

To make these chores easier, make a shopping list in advance and arrange items according to store layout to reduce walking and use less energy. You can also order groceries online or ask a friend or family member to help you shop.

Prioritize easy recipes that don't need much preparation when making meals on low-energy days. Use convenience foods like pre-cut veggies, canned beans, or pre-cooked grains to cut down on cooking time and effort. Batch cooking can save your life—make bigger batches of meals that can be frozen and reheated at a later time. Invest in kitchen appliances like food processors or slow cookers to make meal preparation easier.

Planning and using these strategies will help you grocery shop and prepare meals more efficiently during low-energy times. Set up a station in your kitchen where all the tools and ingredients you'll need are easily accessible. Break down tasks into smaller, manageable steps and take breaks as needed.

Embrace shortcuts like using disposable cookware or pre-portioned ingredients to minimize cleanup.

COMPREHENDING ALLERGIES AND FOOD SENSITIVITIES

Understanding and managing food sensitivities and allergies is crucial for people with chronic fatigue syndrome (CFS) to maintain overall health and manage symptoms. You can track how different foods affect your energy levels and general well-being by keeping a food diary. Common triggers for CFS include gluten, dairy, soy, and certain additives. You can identify specific food sensitivities by working with a registered dietitian or healthcare provider, or you can do allergy testing or elimination diets.

Read food labels carefully before shopping and cooking to avoid allergies or ingredients that could cause symptoms. Prioritize fresh, unprocessed ingredients and choose whole foods whenever possible. Try different ingredients or recipes that can accommodate dietary restrictions without sacrificing flavor or nutrition.

Clearly explain your dietary requirements to loved ones so that meals are prepared safely when you dine together. Educate others and yourself about the significance of food safety and cross-contamination. By taking proactive measures to manage food allergies and sensitivities, you can lessen the symptoms of chronic fatigue syndrome and improve your general health.

EFFECTIVE WAYS FOR FRIENDS AND FAMILY TO SUPPORT NUTRITIONAL NEEDS

When it comes to managing dietary restrictions and chronic fatigue syndrome (CFS), family and friends' support is essential. Begin by telling your loved ones about your unique dietary needs and restrictions; make it clear which foods are safe and which should be avoided because of allergies or sensitivities; promote open communication; and be patient as they adjust to meeting your dietary needs.

When organizing meals or get-togethers, recommend easy recipes that suit your dietary requirements. Offer to supply substitute ingredients or make a dish that everyone will like. If you are hosting, think about having more control over the menu by having the get-togethers at home. If not, pick eateries that provide a variety of menu options or can accommodate special dietary needs.

Share resources with them, such as recipes or articles that can help them better understand CFS and its dietary implications; encourage them to ask questions and seek clarification if they are unsure about food choices or meal preparation techniques; express gratitude for their support and understanding; and recognize the effort they put into accommodating your dietary needs.

Together, you can navigate the challenges of managing chronic fatigue syndrome and create inclusive dining experiences that prioritize health and well-being. By fostering understanding and collaboration, you can create a supportive network that respects your dietary needs while enjoying meaningful social interactions.